Stroke and Brain Injury Unraveled

Prevention, Causes, Symptoms, Diagnosis, Treatment, Recovery and Rehabilitation of One of the Most Debilitating Maladies You Hope You Never Have in Your Lifetime

Arun Thaploo

Copyright © 2015 by Arun Thaploo.

All rights reserved. No portion of this book may be reproduced—mechanically, electronically, or by any other means, including photocopying—without written permission of the author.

Dedication

In the memory of and dedicated to
my dad Avtar Thaploo,
a mentor, a friend, a thinker, and an altruist.

Your FREE gift

I want to show my gratitude for supporting my work. Therefore, I want to give you a gift.

Email me at contactarunthaploo@gmail.com and I will send you a gift as soon as I can. You will receive your gift as a PDF file.

In addition, get notified when I release new books. You will also be notified of occasional special offers on various books and resources.

Contents

Why I Wrote This Book and Why Should You Listen to Me? 1
Why You Should Read This Book? 5
What Am I Going to Cover? 7
Chapter 1 - What is a Stroke? 13
Chapter 2 - What Are the Various Types of Stroke? 17
Chapter 3 - What Causes a Stroke? 21
Chapter 4 - Are You a Candidate for a Stroke? 27
Chapter 5 - How to Identify a Hidden Mini Stroke That Happened in the Past 35
Chapter 6 - How to Recognize the Symptoms of a Major Stroke 41
Chapter 7 - How to Diagnose a Stroke 45
Chapter 8 - How to Treat a Stroke Patient 55
Chapter 9 - How to Prevent Another Stroke in the Near Future 65
Chapter 10 - How Does a Person's Life Change After a Major Stroke 69
Chapter 11 - How to Arrange Treatment and Home Care for a Stroke Patient 81

Epilogue	89
About the Author	91
Other Title by the Author	93
Urgent Plea	95

Why I Wrote This Book and Why Should You Listen to Me?

The human brain has always been an enigma for me. Although I have been intrigued with it since childhood, I started taking a keen interest in studying the human brain in 2006. My focus areas have been the brain's anatomy, creativity, performance, functionality, and the latest brain research. However, I wish I had also focused on various brain diseases and brain disorders, stroke in particular. Circumstances mandated that I pay close attention to stroke in December 2009. That was when my dad suddenly had a stroke. Everyone in the family was flabbergasted, my mom in particular.

I knew that some of the major risk factors for stroke were elevated blood pressure, high levels of cholesterol, smoking, and diabetes. However, my dad did not fit any of these criteria. And here is the irony: While I was growing up, I would barely see my dad getting sick, not even with colds, headaches, or allergies. Moreover, he would not take any over-the-counter medications. He was a vegetarian, never smoked, and never drank. He was extremely healthy all his life until that fateful day of

December 11, 2009. Over the next five years, my dad had several more strokes, including a major one on June 29, 2012, that left him confined to bed. Those five years, particularly the last two and a half years when he was bedridden, were a time of extreme emotional outbursts, pathos, and tenacity for the entire family, especially my mother. My dad left the world for his eternal ethereal abode on November 25, 2014.

As my dad's experience shows, being free of any visible ailments does not necessarily mean that everything is all right with your health. You do not know what is happening deep inside your body. You may have hidden symptoms of some malady about which you are not at all aware. That is why it is imperative to get your physical exams done on a regular basis and to talk to the doctor and your family immediately if you feel some neurological problem at any time.

Before his first stroke, my dad led an incredible life. He firmly believed in the "Pay It Forward" principle and would always be willing to help others in good and bad times. He led a life full of passion, adventure, and purpose. The strokes changed all that. Unfortunately, there was some medical remissness in his treatment from the very beginning as well. I started noticing subtle changes in his personality and thinking after the first few strokes, although his motor skills were still intact.

Living far off from my parents put emotional and mental stress on me. When I could not go see them, I felt like I was dying several times every day. I kept thinking,

"What if something wrong happens again?" or "What if there is a phone call in the middle of the night because my dad had another stroke?" With my heart racing fast, I would wonder, "What if …?"

During a conversation with my dad in January 2012, he told me that I should write a book about stroke. He wanted me to make other people aware of the devastating effects of this malady so that they would benefit from the knowledge. It is my conviction that after reading this book, you will gain enough awareness of stroke to help yourself, your family, and other people you care about, if there is a need.

In the past, strokes were most prevalent in individuals older than 65 years or so. However, the way this disease is spreading in much younger people mandates a deeper soul searching and greater awareness.

Why You Should Read This Book?

I wrote this book keeping "You" the reader in mind and your risks of having a stroke, its prevention, diagnosis, treatment and so on. However, there will be instances where I am assuming that you are a "Caregiver" for a stroke patient. In those scenarios, you will be learning a lot of information about taking the best care of the patient without losing your sanity. The patient could be your family member, a relative or a friend.

This book will be valuable for a novice on stroke and equally useful for a person who has some knowledge of stroke. It is my firm belief that after reading this book and assimilating the contents of this book, it will turn out as one of the best books you have ever read on stroke. This book might save your life or the lives of your dear ones from one of the most agonizing maladies ever known to humankind.

You might be wondering why I said an agonizing malady. I am going to postulate this statement with an analogy. As you may know, the Central Processing Unit (CPU) is like a brain of the computer. The CPU processes most of the instructions and calculations in a computer. If there is something wrong with the CPU, the computer may not work at all. Similarly, the human brain controls all of the functionality of the human body like motor skills, memory, speech, vision, body temperature, heartbeat, breathing, hearing and so on. Any brain injury can have a colossal effect on the body. That is why it is important to keep this invaluable organ enclosed in our skull in top condition.

Let me be very candid here. This book is not for everyone. Because if you are not serious about keeping your brain healthy or if you do not care, then I guess this is one of the thousands of health books out there. You might read it and after some time just forget about the material.

However if you are extremely serious about your brain health and want to live an active life as long as you are alive, then this book is for you. It is for people who care about themselves or their loved ones. It is for individuals who can visualize the debilitating effects of brain damage and prevent it from happening in the first place. It is for people who are farsighted, empathetic, and have a clarity in life.

What Am I Going to Cover?

This chapter will give you a quick snapshot of what I am going to cover in this book. Each paragraph corresponds to a chapter.

The first chapter will teach you what a stroke is and give you some statistics of this enervating disease. It will also teach you when a stroke is a medical emergency and why you should seek immediate medical attention. You will gain insight into what can happen if the symptoms remain unaddressed as time flies, or if you take the warning signs in a casual manner.

The second chapter will cover various types of strokes and their subtypes. You will learn about the Transient Ischemic Attacks (TIA) in particular. TIAs are also referred to as silent strokes as often times people cannot identify their symptoms. Normally it does not affect your motor skills and it is a very subtle type of stroke.

The third chapter will give you detailed information about the various causes of stroke. You will learn about the most common forms of stroke and why ischemic strokes are more pronounced than hemorrhagic strokes.

The fourth chapter will elaborate on whether you are a candidate for a stroke. It will list most of the common causes of the likelihood of having a stroke in case you have one or more of these preexisting conditions. The intent is to warn you in advance so that you can take a corrective course and preempt the chances of having a stroke.

The fifth chapter has an unusual significance, and you should pay close attention to the contents of this chapter. It will give you information about some of the symptoms that you might be facing right at this moment that most of the people often overlook. Being mindful about these subtle symptoms will go a long way in averting a major stroke in the future, especially after you cross your 65th birthday.

The sixth chapter will delve into making you understand the symptoms of a major stroke. It means how to recognize that you already had a major stroke or a stroke is underway right now at this very moment. You will learn about various self-tests that you can run on yourself at that point. Assuming you have not lost consciousness due to a severe stroke. You can also run these tests on a family member or on a person who is beside you if you notice these symptoms in them. Once there is a confirmation of a stroke, you should avail emergency medical help immediately. Many precious lives can be saved if individuals are well-informed about these simple tests. I know people who did not have a clue of what was going on when one of their family members was having a stroke. They were just massaging the family member's arms and legs as the patient had been complaining of numbness in the arms and legs.

The seventh chapter will teach you the diagnosis of a stroke at a doctor's office in detail. You will learn about various tests the doctor might recommend before starting a treatment plan. It is another important chapter in this book, and you should learn the material in this chapter and commit the information to memory if you can. One of the distinctive features of this chapter is that it will give you information about many blood tests that you can get at the doctor's office. Many people suffer from strokes due to various blood disorders. These blood tests will rule out any issues with your blood. You will also learn about various tests recommended for the brain and the heart as well.

The eighth chapter is all about the treatment after a person has had a stroke. You will learn about what medicines the doctor might recommend. You will also learn about what surgeries and procedures the doctor might recommend, depending upon the type of stroke and the severity level of the stroke. Both the ischemic and hemorrhagic strokes will be covered in detail.

The ninth chapter assumes that, unfortunately, you or your loved one have already had one stroke in the past. Now how can you prevent the likelihood of having another stroke? However, keep in mind that certain patients can get repetitive strokes in the future due to certain medical conditions. Some other reasons being a wrong diagnosis, invasive tests done after having the first stroke, or not getting treatment on time after having the first major stroke. This chapter will also throw some light on how to channel your thoughts toward empowerment and look ahead to life. You will get tips on coming out stronger after you survived a stroke and how to enhance your emotional and mental energy levels. You will also learn about how to develop that enthusiasm, purpose and love for life despite suffering from a stroke in the past.

The tenth chapter will discuss how a person's life changes after suffering either a major or a minor stroke. I will cover the emotional and mental ordeals a stroke patient might go through besides the physical and cognitive deficits in particular. For example, how a person who has had a fearless personality all his life might start becoming fearful. How there might be frequent mood swings in a stroke patient or how as a caregiver you might feel so powerless and even cry out of despair. Just internalize the sufferings in consonance with the emotional and mental trauma faced by a stroke survivor while reading this chapter. Your heart will bleed for that person.

Finally, the eleventh chapter will give you information about how to arrange treatment and homecare for a stroke patient. Besides outlining the things that you will have to purchase for the patient, it will also cover the correct methodologies of handling a stroke patient from the caregiver's perspective. While caring for the stroke patient, I want you to understand the stressful aspects of attending to the patient's daily needs. You will learn about how to minimize the stress to a manageable level. Remember, if a person suffers from a long-term disability, it takes a colossal toll on the entire family, friends and extended family.

All right, so while paying close attention to the material covered in the book, let us get started.

Chapter 1

What is a Stroke?

Before we get started on stroke, here are some startling facts. Every year more than 15 million people suffer a stroke worldwide. Around 10 million die and another 5 million are left permanently disabled. It is the second leading cause of death worldwide above the age of 65 years and the fourth leading cause of death in the United States. Imagine how the life of an individual changes after a stroke. For example, a person can suffer from paralysis, loss of memory, loss of speech, confusion and difficulty in thinking, vision problems, inability to swallow, partially or entirely dependent on others, etc.

Imagine a person who spent so many years of his life learning languages, wisdom, personal experiences and sweet memories lose them in no time due to a stroke. Visualize a person who lost his speech due to a stroke and who is unable to express himself. For example, talk about how he is feeling, his pain and agonies, and so on. Do you relate to such person's disparity?

This book is not an authoritative guide on stroke as neuroscience is an evolving field. Besides, brain scientists and researchers are coming out with new findings every year. However, this book will give you enough information to understand how to stay well-informed about this appalling disease, and I am going to explain it in a non-professional's language.

If a person has had a massive stroke, it could either kill the person or make the person bedridden for the rest of his life. Some people may recover partially after a stroke and have limited motor skills thereafter. While some people who are fortunate enough may recover almost completely after a prolonged treatment and through physical therapy. However, the most unfortunate part is that some people who have had a massive stroke lose all their cognitive skills within no time. Just visualize the mental and emotional state of the patient.

Our brain needs a constant supply of blood and oxygen for optimum health and perform various motor functions. In fact, even though our brains weigh only 2% of our total weight, it needs around 35% of oxygen. A stroke occurs if there is a restriction of oxygen-rich blood to a particular area of the brain. Within a few minutes, the brain cells start to die in the affected area. Unfortunately, the brain cells that die do not regenerate.

An individual will start seeing the symptoms in the part of the body that the damaged cells were controlling. If the stroke is massive, the patient will begin noticing the symptoms immediately. For example, signs of a droopy face, slurred speech, sudden weakness in arms and legs particularly on one side of the body, utter confusion to think or understand. He may also notice acute and very different kind of headache with a possibility of vomiting. Other symptoms like paralysis on one side of the body or both (inability to move freely), facial paralysis, vision impairments, are also common. In some cases, the stroke might be temporary without even the person realizing it (Transient Ischemic Attack).

A stroke can be a very serious medical condition and in those situations, every minute counts. If not treated immediately a stroke can cause death, long-term disability or even a permanent brain damage.

There is an acronym that you need to remember called FAST. You will learn more about this acronym in "How to Recognize the Symptoms of a Major Stroke" chapter. In the meantime, just remember FAST stands for "Face Arm Speech Time". Remember this acronym and spread the word in your family and among people you care about.

Keep in mind that the first four hours are extremely critical in treating a stroke patient. Many complications can be avoided if the patient is given immediate medical attention. It will reduce damage to the patient's brain and in most cases prevent long-term disabilities. In fact, if the first stroke is treated within the first four hours, it can reduce the chances of having another stroke in some patients in the near future.

Besides, it is very crucial to talk to a family member immediately if you are experiencing symptoms of a stroke so that the family member can arrange for a medical emergency. Do not withhold these symptoms to yourself thinking that if you talk about it to family members, they will just freak out or start crying. They will get more distressed if you do not tell them about your symptoms and something terribly wrong happens to your health later on. If you are alone in a particular situation but able to talk, call 911 immediately if you are in the US, or the corresponding emergency number in your country.

Chapter 2

What Are the Various Types of Stroke?

There are three types of stroke and each type of stroke can have different caveats. Each type of stroke can occur in different areas of the brain resulting in different symptoms and consequences.

1) Ischemic Stroke
2) Hemorrhagic Stroke
3) Transient Ischemic Attack (TIA)

Let us get started with each type of stroke. Incidentally, the ischemic stroke and hemorrhagic stroke are further divided into two main types.

1) Ischemic Stroke:
It is the most common form of stroke and around 80% strokes fall into this category. An ischemic stroke can occur when the blood vessel carrying oxygen-rich blood to the brain is obstructed by a blood clot. It results in the blood not reaching that part of the brain and damaging

the brain cells in that area.

Here are the two types of ischemic stroke:

Thrombotic Stroke

A thrombotic stroke is caused by a blood clot (medical term - thrombus) that forms inside one of the arteries which supplies oxygenated blood to the brain. The clot remains at the site of its formation and blood flow is obstructed. The blood clot itself can be of two types: Large Vessel Thrombosis (LVT) and Small Vessel Thrombosis (SVT). The large vessel thrombosis occurs in the brain's larger arteries. The small vessel thrombosis occurs in the small arterial blood vessel, and this type of stroke is called Lacunar Infarction. It is also called Cryptogenic stroke because the possible causes cannot be easily identified. Even undergoing various tests might not give an insight to what caused the stroke.

Embolic Stroke

In an embolic stroke, a blood clot, a fatty material, or plaque travels through the bloodstream all the way to an artery in the brain. When the clot travels further down to a blood vessel narrow enough to block its path downstream, an embolic stroke occurs. In other words, that specific part of the brain tissue further down the blood clot gets damaged due to lack of oxygen-rich blood.

2) Hemorrhagic Stroke:

These types of strokes are less common and around 20% of strokes fall into this category. Brain arteries bursting open (aneurysm burst) or a weakened blood vessel leak cause hemorrhagic strokes. The blood leakage spreads into and around the brain, creating brain swelling and pressure, which results in cell and tissue damage in the brain.

Here are the two types of hemorrhagic stroke:

Intracerebral Hemorrhage:

It is the most common form of hemorrhagic stroke. It is caused by a leakage in a blood vessel inside the brain. The leaked blood spreads into the adjacent area of the affected part of the brain. The bleeding results in the death of brain cells and the affected area of the brain stops functioning properly.

Subarachnoid Hemorrhage:

Bleeding can occur when the blood vessel on the surface of the brain bursts open. This condition is known as aneurysm burst. This bleeding occurs between the inner and middle layers of the membranes that cover the brain. In other words, bleeding occurs in an area between the brain and the tissue covering the brain.

3) Transient Ischemic Attack (TIA):

TIAs are different from the other two types of stroke discussed earlier. In a TIA, the blood flow to a part of the brain is stopped temporarily, usually few minutes to few hours. After that, the symptoms disappear, and the person recovers immediately from that point forward. TIAs are somewhat similar to ischemic strokes in the sense that they are caused by blood clots or plaque buildup in the body. TIAs are also referred as "warning strokes" as they may suggest that a far more severe stroke is about to happen in the near future. Therefore, this type of stroke should also be treated as a medical emergency. However, here is an irony: Many times TIAs are unnoticed by individuals. The reason being that a person does not experience a dramatic impediment in his motor skills or cognition.

Chapter 3

What Causes a Stroke?

There are different reasons for various types of stroke, although the causes of ischemic stroke and Transient Ischemic Attack (TIA) are somewhat similar. So ischemic stroke and TIA will be covered together, followed by hemorrhagic stroke. Let us learn more about them in detail.

Ischemic Stroke and Transient Ischemic Attack: As mentioned in the last chapter, this is the most common type of stroke as around 80% of strokes fall into this category. Many medical conditions increase the risk of ischemic stroke. Let me reiterate, an ischemic stroke or a TIA is caused due to plaque buildup in any of the arteries in the body. It results in the oxygenated blood not reaching the brain. The plaque can build in arteries that run into the brain, the neck or even in the heart.

There is a condition called atherosclerosis that results in fats, cholesterol and other substances depositing on the inner walls of the arteries. With the passage of time, this fatty substance called plaque hardens, and it narrows down the arteries of either the brain, neck or the heart. The major ramifications of this abnormal behavior result in limiting the supply of blood to the brain.

However, the plaque buildup does not happen in days or months. In most cases, it takes years and years for the plaque to be deposited in the arteries, without the affected person knowing about it. Moreover, age is also a reason for the plaque to accumulate on the inner walls of the arteries. So, the more inflammation in the body, the more chances of plaque buildup in the arteries. That is why it is a good idea to get the inflammation test done periodically to find out how much the body is inflamed. The test is called a Sedimentation Rate Test, and you will find more information about this test in the diagnostics chapter.

Sometimes atherosclerosis can also form small lesions in the brain. These lesions may form in the small arteries of the brain that can restrict the blood flow to the brain.

Once massive plaque builds up in an artery, it might crack or rupture sometimes and cause injury to the artery. However, the disc-shaped cells called blood platelets stick to the area of the injured artery. With the result, a lump is formed to seal the ruptured area. Once blood coagulates near the affected area completely, it results in the formation of blood clots. These clots can sometimes partially or entirely block an artery.

The plaque can develop in any artery of the body, including the three most important organs namely the brain, heart, and neck. The two arteries that run on the left and right side of the neck are called carotid arteries.

These arteries are responsible for supplying oxygen-rich blood to the brain, face, scalp and the neck. When a significant amount of plaque builds up in the carotid arteries, the symptom is called the carotid artery disease. Carotid artery disease is a leading cause of many ischemic strokes and TIAs all across the globe. Therefore, pay special attention to protect your neck from any significant injury.

One of the best things that you can do to protect neck injury is not to sleep on your stomach. When you sleep on your stomach, you have to turn your head to the side to breathe. It can result in an unnecessary tension on your neck, spine and incidentally your carotid arteries. Even if you are working with a renounced chiropractor for your sprains and pain, you should avoid any major adjustments to your neck. I have heard about a few cases where people have suffered from strokes after getting their neck adjustments from a chiropractor.

Now let us consider another scenario. Imagine a piece of plaque or a piece of blood clot breaking away from the wall of an artery. This blood clot or a piece of plaque can be released from any artery in any part of the body. If this piece of clot or plaque travels through the blood stream all the way to an artery of the brain and is stuck, there is an immediate restriction of blood supply to that part of the brain. The brain cells and tissues near the affected area are instantly damaged. This type of ischemic stroke is called an embolic stroke as you learned in the previous chapter.

Some other reasons for getting an ischemic stroke are

due to various disorders of the blood and due to varying heart conditions resulting in a blood clot formation. As an example, atrial fibrillation is a type of embolic stroke. In arterial fibrillation, the upper chambers of the heart contract in a very fast and asymmetrical way. As a result, some blood is accumulated in the heart chambers. This excess blood in one of the chambers of the heart can lead to a blood clot formation. That is why it is important to evaluate your heart for irregular heartbeats. A comprehensive Holter monitor test can evaluate irregular heartbeats. You will find more information about this test in the "How to diagnose a stroke" chapter.

Hemorrhagic Stroke:

When there is a sudden bleeding in the brain of an individual, it means the person has had a hemorrhagic stroke. The bleeding results in brain swelling and the pressure inside the skull increases. The reason being that the brain does not have any room for expansion as it is enclosed within the skull. The swelling and the pressure further damage the brain cells and tissues. At the time of a hemorrhagic stroke, the individual will have a chronic and painful headache. This headache is different from an ordinary headache or even a migraine headache. It is intense and unbearable. As an analogy, it will sound as if some sharp objects are pierced into the skull of the individual.

The common causes of hemorrhagic stroke are high blood pressure, Aneurysms and Arteriovenous Malformations. Let us discuss them one by one.

High Blood Pressure: What is blood pressure? It is the force with which the blood pushes against the walls of the arteries as the heart pumps blood to all parts of the body. If the blood pressure stays high for a prolonged time and the individual keeps overlooking the symptoms, it can have a devastating effect on the entire body. The brain can have a hemorrhagic stroke if a person's blood pressure stays high for a long time. In fact, people with high blood pressure have a stroke risk of four to six times greater than those with normal blood pressure.

Aneurysms: Aneurysms are balloon shaped bulges in an artery. If you fill a balloon with air and keep pumping air into it after it has reached its threshold, what will happen? It will pop immediately. The same thing happens when an individual is suffering from an aneurysm. These faulty arteries and veins can rupture within the brain, resulting in a hemorrhagic stroke. Things are exacerbated if people with aneurysm also have high blood pressure.

Arteriovenous Malformation: An AVM is a twist of abnormal blood vessels connecting arteries and veins in the brain. As you might know, the arteries are responsible for transporting oxygen-rich blood from the heart to the brain, and the veins are responsible for carrying oxygen-starved blood back to the lungs and the heart. If a person is suffering from AVM, the normal functionality of the arteries and veins is disrupted due to the knot between the two. This condition can result in a hemorrhagic stroke. However, the good thing is that people with AVM are present in less than 1% of the population, and people are generally born with them. Some people can develop it later in their lives. Individuals who get frequent seizures and headaches should be diagnosed for these symptoms. If AVM is diagnosed early, it can be treated successfully to prevent brain damage or stroke.

Chapter 4

Are You a Candidate for a Stroke?

Here are some of the risk factors for getting a stroke in your lifetime. It is not an exhaustive list, but they are the main causes of getting a stroke.

Blood Disorder: The quality of blood flowing in your circulatory system has an enormous role to play in your overall well-being, including your brain health. The blood should be neither too thin nor too thick. If your blood is too thick, then there are chances of clot formation that can cause an ischemic stroke. If your blood is too thin and you have weak arteries, there are chances of a hemorrhagic stroke.

High Cholesterol: If you have high levels of cholesterol and triglycerides, then that is a risk factor for a stroke. An example of a stroke due to high Low-density lipoprotein (LDL) Cholesterol levels is called Large Vessel Thrombosis. It is a type of thrombotic stroke that you learned in the "Various types of Stroke" chapter. That is why you should keep your cholesterol level within a normal range.

High blood pressure: This is another major reason for a stroke, especially a thrombotic stroke that is a type of ischemic stroke. The Small Vessel Thrombotic stroke primarily happens due to high blood pressure. If your blood pressure stays constantly higher than 140/90 mmHg, you have a risk factor for stroke.

Diabetes: If you are diabetic, you should be extra careful about your health. An individual who has diabetes can face a far worse condition after a stroke than people who are not diabetic. Nature has given us an astonishing mechanism for wellness and self-healing. Sometimes, when there is a blockage in an artery and the oxygen supply is interrupted, other arteries can usually deliver the oxygen by bypassing the blockage. However, people with diabetes can get affected with atherosclerosis about which you learned in the previous chapter. In such a condition, many of the bypass arteries are blocked as well, thus preventing the oxygen supply to the brain. Eventually, this condition can lead to a stroke.

Heart Disease: A person having a major heart disease, for example, coronary artery disease, heart failure, etc. has a greater chance of getting a stroke. If there is plaque buildup in the heart, or if there is a high level of inflammation in the heart, chances of clot formation in the heart are high. If this clot travels all the way to the brain, it can cause a stroke.

Arterial Fibrillation (AF): A person suffering from arterial fibrillation can be at a risk of having a stroke. In AF, there is a problem with the rate of rhythm of the heartbeat. The heart of a person who is suffering from AF beats too quickly, too slowly, or irregularly. Disorganized electrical signals in the two upper chambers of the heart called "Atrium" are the main cause of fibrillation of the heart. Sometimes people may be unaware of the symptoms of AF. However, AF increases the risk of having a stroke and can even result in a heart failure in certain cases. Arterial fibrillation can be recorded and studied using an electronic device called a Holter monitor.

Family History: There is some correlation between stroke and family history, but not in all the cases, and that is a good news. If your parent or a grandparent has had a stroke especially before age 65, you are also likely to share some of the risk factors. Although making formidable lifestyle changes and continually monitoring your health profile mitigates that risk.

Brain Aneurysms: They are balloon-like bulges in a blood vessel that can stretch and burst under pressure in the brain causing a stroke. Unfortunately, sometimes they are hard to diagnose until they rupture.

Head and Neck Injury: Any major injury to the head or neck can result in some strokes as well. An injury to the head can cause internal bleeding of the brain, resulting in a hemorrhagic stroke. Likewise, an injury to the neck can lead to a tearing of the vertebrae or damage to the carotid arteries. Sometimes an ischemic stroke can take place due to sudden elongation or twisting of the neck, especially in old people. As mentioned earlier, there are some risks associated with the improper manipulation of the neck at a chiropractor's office as well.

Age and Gender: If you are 65 years and above, then the chances of stroke are more pronounced. After age 75, the risks are even higher. However, it does not mean that a younger person cannot have a stroke. But the older you are, the higher the risk. People over 65 have a seven-fold greater risk of dying from a stroke than the general population. At younger ages, men are more likely to have a stroke than women are. However, at an advanced age, women are more likely to get a stroke than men are.

Race and Ethnicity: Strokes are more prevalent in Alaska natives, African American, and American Indians adults than Caucasian, Hispanic or Asian Americans in the United States before 65 years of age. However, after age 65 this tendency is less pronounced.

Excessive alcohol consumption: If you are a heavy drinker, you are at an increased risk of having a stroke. So either give up alcohol consumption or drink in moderation.

Smoking and Tobacco use: Like drinking, heavy smokers have a higher risk of having a stroke. When you smoke, the amount of oxygen that reaches your cells and tissues decreases. Besides, smoking damages the blood vessels and the lungs. And the damaged blood vessels can rupture, resulting in a stroke.

Certain drugs and medicines: People can also have a stroke by consuming certain drugs and medicines, e.g., cocaine, amphetamines, etc. Therefore, it is important to read about the side effects of specific drugs and medicines before taking them.

Anxiety and Depression: People who are constantly anxious or suffering chronic depression may have a stroke as well. Some doctors say that during extreme and prolonged bouts of anxiety, the blood pressure can spike up suddenly, and that can cause a stroke. However, there is still a lot of research going on regarding this subject. Therefore, there is no concrete evidence that can suggest a correlation between depression and stroke.

Lack of physical activity or having a sedentary lifestyle: If you have a sedentary way of life, your chances of having a stroke increase. By sitting most of the time, the blood circulation in the body, especially your legs and butt, does not happen properly. Months and months of inactivity can cause muscle cramps, sciatic nerve problems, and varicose veins in the legs. A sedentary lifestyle can also result in circulatory problems and thus increase the chances of stroke. So keep moving and avoid sitting for too long.

An extreme amount of worrying and excessive thinking: Extreme levels of worrying for years and years can also result in symptoms of a stroke. Besides, people who think too much also have a risk of stroke. One of the reasons cited by researchers and doctors is that a habitual heavy-thinker is straining his brain considerably over a long period of time. It results in changes in the brain's composition if the trend continues for years and years. Eventually, it can cause a stroke in some cases.

Unhealthy diet: What you eat can also have a bearing

on your brain health. Prolonged consumption of an unhealthy diet can also accelerate the chances of getting a stroke. Unhealthy food can inflame your body, raise your cholesterol and triglycerides levels, raise your sugar levels, increase your blood pressure, etc.

Overweight and Obesity: People who are overweight have a higher risk of having a stroke. The more weight an individual has, the more blood vessels are present in the body, and the harder the heart has to work to pump blood out to the entire body. Hence, if there is a buildup of plaque in the arteries, there are chances of the plaque breaking up. Subsequently, that can lead to a clot formation, and if the clot gets closer to the brain, it can cause a stroke.

Other Medical Conditions: Certain medical conditions like Vasculitis, Cerebral Amyloid Angiopathy, and Bleeding Disorders can cause a stroke. Vasculitis is a condition that results in the inflammation of blood vessels due to an internal infection, medicine, or other diseases. Cerebral Amyloid Angiopathy is a type of angiopathy (a disease of the blood vessels), resulting in the deposition of amyloids in the walls of the blood vessels of the nervous system. Amyloids are an insoluble fibrous protein that deposits in the inner walls of the blood vessels in the brain. In a person with an extremely high level of Cerebral Amyloid Angiopathy, the protein deposits can cause the blood vessel walls to crack. In that case, blood can leak out and damage the brain, resulting in a hemorrhagic stroke.

Cerebral Amyloid Angiopathy is not a new disease.

However, in the last few years, neurologists have come to know a little more about it and the role it plays in hemorrhagic strokes. In some cases, it is the cause of dementia in patients. Some neurosurgeons sometimes even suggest a brain biopsy to evaluate it further. To consider something like that, one needs to understand the pros and cons of doing a brain biopsy. Most doctors do not recommend it.

Chapter 5

How to Identify a Hidden Mini Stroke That Happened in the Past

This chapter will give you information about recognizing the subtle symptoms of neurological issues that you may be facing right now. Most of the people will overlook these symptoms due to ignorance or leading a fast-paced lifestyle or having the "Do not care" attitude. So please pay special attention to this chapter.

Be mindful and immediately see your doctor if you observe any unusual behavior of your motor skills. A qualified doctor should evaluate these symptoms, especially if the symptoms are repetitive.

So let us get started:

1) Lately, have you noticed that you make many typing mistakes on your smartphone, computer, or tablet? For example, you want to press the letter "o", but your finger taps the letter "i". On the other hand, you want to type the letter "j", but your finger involuntarily moves to "g". Besides, this behavior has been consistent for several weeks

or several months now, even though you have never experienced this peculiar behavior before.

2) You take a shower in the morning, and you are about to come out of the bathtub. While you lift your leg to step out of the bathtub, your foot hits the edge of the bathtub, and you get hurt. You wonder what went wrong as you swung your leg the right way while coming out of the bathtub. I would highly recommend you maintain a journal and notate these incidents. Write the approximate time and frequency of these events.

3) You try to close a door and raise your arm to grab the doorknob, but instead, your hand hits the edge of the door and your hand gets hurt.

4) You get up early in the morning from bed, and you notice some body-imbalance while taking your first few steps. Sometimes you have to grab the doorknob or get support from the wall to maintain your balance.

5) Sometimes do you feel that when you are thinking, you cannot think clearly? For example, you cannot process information succinctly and with ease, as you used to in the past.

6) If you were ever diagnosed with Portal Vein Thrombosis, you have a high risk of developing a stroke. Immediately consult a neurologist to evaluate it further. Sometimes a person suffering from Portal Vein Thrombosis can have a stroke several years after the thrombosis. Check with your doctor if taking a baby aspirin once a day might be something to consider.

7) Have you realized that you cannot remember simple

things or some new information, even though you are trying hard to remember it? Pay particular attention to your short-term memory. For example, you learn some new information and then you try to commit it to memory by being mindful and through repetition. However, after a few days you forget about what you had learned. If it happens too often and your family members start questioning your memory, you should get yourself evaluated by a qualified doctor. However, there are some exceptions. As people start aging, it is okay to forget sometimes, as it is part of the aging brain. This is particularly true if you are not strengthening your memory with everyday problem solving, puzzles, eating brain health foods, and leading an active lifestyle.

8) Watch out for frequent dizziness when you are walking or standing for too long. It is also called a vertigo. Even too much of neck twisting and lying down on a couch while reading for hours and hours can create neurological problems later on. For example, reading for long while lying down on a couch without proper head support can result in spondylitis. In fact, it can also affect your carotid arteries.

9) Have you started observing that when you talk, and you want to say a particular word, a different word comes out of your mouth? For example, you wish to say something like, "So you want to grab the car key," but when you verbalize the sentence, a different word comes out of your mouth. For example, "So you want to grab the far key?" If you pay attention, you might realize that you

are making more of these mistakes. Moreover, all of this is happening automatically. In the end, you feel very puzzled and embittered. If you are talking in a formal gathering or giving a presentation, these mistakes might even embarrass you.

10) Do you feel a burning sensation emanating from your arms, legs, hands, neck, and feet continually? Or maybe a sensation of tingling (a feeling of pins and needles). In medical terms, it is known as paresthesia. It can be caused by an injury to the nerves or due to pinched nerves. Prolonged burning sensation of the arm can also be a sign of multiple sclerosis. Your immune system attacks the protective sheath that covers your nerves in this disease. Moreover, an intense burning sensation in the arm, particularly when it happens suddenly and on one side of the body, can be a symptom of a stroke or a heart attack.

11) Have you been feeling constant numbness in your arms and legs for months and months? It can probably happen due to damage to the nerves that come out of the neck toward the arms and hands. Another reason could be Thoracic Outlet Syndrome, which is caused by compression of the nerves or blood vessels in the thoracic outlet. It is an area between the base of the neck and armpit, including the chest and the front of the shoulders. There is a test that is called Nerve Conduction Study (NCS), which might be recommended by your doctor. This test measures how correctly and how fast the nerves send electrical signals to various parts of the body. It is a

very useful test to evaluate various problems with the peripheral nervous system.

12) If you are not moving your arms and legs frequently, you will have a higher risk of getting a stroke in the near future, compared to people who exercise and do not have a sedentary lifestyle. There is sufficient data available to prove this point in the medical field. People who sit most of the time develop more blood clots than people who have high energy and are active most of the time.

13) Don't think too much on unnecessary things. Although the sentence is very subtle, the meaning is very profound. If you keep thinking most of the time, you are tiring your brain enormously. That is not good for your brain health. In fact, if you keep thinking and worrying all the time, it will become a new habit. Your brain will realize that it is okay to think all the time. With the result, it will put too much pressure on the brain and eventually do a colossal damage to your mental well-being. Too much thinking will also impact your memory power, your focus, and your alertness. Sometimes, I tell people metaphorically that you should assume that you have no brain in your head some times during the day. And that might probably help some people who are thinking most of the time. You should also explore and implement various relaxation techniques for your body and mind from time to time. It can help in reducing wavering thoughts in the mind and increase mental alertness.

Here is the last point, one that I wanted to leave for the end. Pay close attention to this paragraph. In some cases, the above symptoms are signs of a Transient Ischemic Attack / Lacunar Infarcts. Most of these attacks happen silently without the person realizing it. During a TIA, the motor skills of an individual do not get drastically impacted; he takes these things very lightly. If there is an impairment of motor skills during a TIA, the person might think that he is getting some temporary numbness due to exertion or something. Once the effects of TIA disappear within minutes or hours, the person thinks he is feeling better again.

Sometimes, when an individual has had a major stroke, the CT Scans/MRIs show previous TIAs and / or Lacunar Infarcts. If the patient had remained extremely vigilant about these abnormal symptoms and taken immediate action, in all likelihood, a major stroke could have been averted. These types of major health issues happen because the individual had not been paying any attention to some of those trivial and often overlooked symptoms as mentioned earlier in this chapter.

So, what is the cure? The best thing you can do is to consult a renowned neurologist, explain your symptoms in detail and follow the doctor's advice.

Chapter 6

How to Recognize the Symptoms of a Major Stroke

The information in this chapter will go a long way in treating a major stroke or a recurrence of a stroke. You should commit the material learned in this chapter to memory. You never know when this information might be useful for you or one of your loved ones.

I will extrapolate a little more about the acronym FAST that was discussed in an earlier chapter.

F stands for Face: Check if a person who you think might be having a stroke has a droopy face. Ask the person to smile and notice for any asymmetry on her face. For example, do you see the lips being uncoordinated? Notice if one side of the lips is lower than the other side.

A stands for Arm: Ask the person to raise her arm and hold it parallel to the ground. Can the person hold on to her arm for as long as you tell her? Notice for any significant tremors in her arm, or if the individual is unable to hold her arm for too long.

S stands for Smile: Ask the person to smile. Can she follow your instructions? Pay close attention to the facial muscles. Also, check the person's eyes. Ask her to blink her eyes several times.

T stands for Time: Remember you need to act fast when you observe the symptoms of stroke. The first four hours are extremely critical in case of a major stroke. Hours of delay in treating the patient can be life-threatening or do colossal damage to the brain and its functionality. If a stroke patient is left untreated for more than four hours, several things can happen. First, a severe stroke can result in the death of an individual, or it can permanently damage some of the functionalities of the brain.

Besides the above FAST test, you can also ask the person to do the following:

- Say a short sentence and ask the person to repeat it. If you notice a slur in her speech or some gibberish, then you know that it is an indication of a stroke.

- Ask the person to open her mouth and observe her tongue. If her tongue is twisted or bent, then you know that something is wrong.

- Watch for sudden, severe, and different types of headaches with no known cause. Remember, when a person is having a massive stroke, she is experiencing chronic headaches on either one side or the entire head.

If the stroke is very severe, then some of the following things can happen.

The patient will lose sensation on a part of her body. For example, a part of the body will be partially paralyzed. The person may not be able to stand up, walk, or move the arms. A person might lose her speech, or she might complain about impairment of vision.

In certain cases, after a complex and severe stroke, a person might lose consciousness and may not be in a position to give her consent for treatment. Therefore, the family members will have to take a decision about the immediate treatment and long-term treatment plans.

When you observe any of these symptoms, immediately call 911 (in USA) or 999 (in United Kingdom). Remember, the first four hours are extremely critical for a person who had a stroke. Treating the patient within the first four hours of a stroke can prevent severe brain damage, or the debilitating symptoms can be even reversed. Always remember, if there is brain damage, the cells in the affected area die and they do not regenerate.

So rather than repenting later, better act swiftly in case you or your loved one is having a stroke, and remember the word FAST.

Chapter 7

How to Diagnose a Stroke

A stroke can be diagnosed based on a variety of symptoms found in the patient. For example, by physically examining the patient's body, running some tests, and studying the patient's medical history including family history.

If the patient is conscious, the doctor may ask the patient or a family member various questions. For example, when and how the symptoms started, any history of high blood pressure, heart disease, family history of stroke, etc.

Next, during the physical exam, the doctor will check the motor skills of the patient and her mental alertness, coordination, and balance. He may check for numbness in various parts of her body, weakness in the face, speech impairments, vision, sensation in the arms and legs, commotion, and cognitive skills.

Once the doctor has completed the physical exam and understood the family history of the patient, he may order some tests. If the condition is severe, the tests will be ordered immediately. The tests that may be ordered fall in three different categories:

A) Tests done on the brain
B) Tests done on the heart
C) Various Blood Tests

Let us discuss the various types of tests in detail:

A) Tests recommended for the brain:

1) A CT Scan: A CT scan uses high radiation X-Rays to take clear pictures of the brain. It is one of the first tests to be performed if it is suspected a stroke may be present. A CT scan can show clear pictures of bleeding in the brain and damage to the brain cells. It is a faster test than an MRI, and may be the first line of action in case of a trauma.

2) A Brain MRI: This test uses magnets and radio waves to create pictures of the brain tissue. It produces better images of the soft tissue of the brain than a CT scan. Thus, it gives more details of the brain tissue and is more sensitive to the abnormalities of the brain.

3) MR Angiography: This test examines the blood vessels in various parts of the body like, brain, neck, heart, legs, pelvis, etc. Sometimes a contrast material, for example, administering iodine produces better pictures of various blood vessels in the body. It is an important test to check for stenosis (abnormal narrowing of a blood vessel) or a brain aneurysm.

4) CT Angiography: This test uses a CT scanner to produce detailed images of both blood vessels and tissues in the brain. In this test, there is an injection of a contrast material in the body through a small catheter placed in a vein. The advantage of CT Angiography over MR Angiography is that it provides precise details about the small blood vessels.

5) **Carotid Artery Ultrasound test:** This test reveals if there is any narrowing or bulging of the carotid artery that could be preventing the flow of oxygen-rich blood to the brain. Part of this test might also include a Doppler ultrasound that can show the speed and direction of the blood traversing through the blood vessels by bouncing high-frequency sound waves (ultrasound) off circulating red blood cells.

6) **Carotid Artery Angiography:** In this test, the doctor inserts a small tube called a catheter through an artery in the groin (femoral artery). To get a clear picture of the artery on the X-Ray, a contrast substance in injected into the tube. The tube is then slowly moved up into one of the carotid arteries. The X-Ray images can then be evaluated to recommend a treatment plan.

B) Tests recommended for the heart:

1) **Electrocardiogram (EKG):** This test gives information about the heart's electrical activity. This test can provide information about pulse rate and whether the pulses are steady or irregular. An EKG can give information about the heart problems that may have resulted in a stroke.

2) **Echocardiogram or Transthoracic Echocardiogram (TTE):** An Echocardiogram is a cardiac ultrasound that uses sound waves to give detailed information about the overall health of your heart. The purpose of this test is to analyze all the four chambers of the heart. This test also investigates the condition of the heart valves, and the aorta that is the largest artery in the body that carries oxygen-rich blood to the entire body. It is a crucial test to detect the probable blood clots in the heart, thinning of the wall of the heart muscle. This test can also give information about blood leaking backward through the heart valves (regurgitation) and decreased blood flow through a heart valve (stenosis).

3) **Holter Monitor:** This is a type of electrocardiogram (EKG) machine that an individual wears for at least 24 hours to continuously record the heart's rhythm. This test is recommended because sometimes during an electrocardiogram test irregular heartbeats are not observed in a patient during that test. An individual may carry the monitor in a pocket, or a pouch worn around the neck. While wearing the monitor, it is important to keep a log of all the activities you do during the entire period. For example, if you exercised, how you felt at a particular time, when you slept and how long, what you ate and at what time, etc. After the stipulated timeframe, the individual returns the monitor to the doctor's office for evaluation. After that, the doctor will look for any abnormal heart rhythms.

C) Tests recommended for the blood:

The following are some of the necessary blood tests the doctor might order. The idea is to understand the quality of blood in the patient. If some of the parameters are out of range, it needs an intervention by the doctor's office.

1) Prothrombin Time: Used to evaluate how long it takes the blood to clot. Standard Range 11.5 - 11.1 seconds

2) Partial Thromboplastin Time: This is another blood test that measures the time it takes your blood to clot - Standard Range 24.0 - 36.0 seconds

3) INR: It stands for International Normalized Ratio. This test evaluates the thickness or the thinness of a person's blood. Standard Range 0.9 - 1.2

4) Homocysteine: It is one of the 20 amino acids that the body requires to synthesize all body protein. If it is present in high strengths, it can be linked to an increased risk of heart attacks and stroke. Standard Range - 3.7 - 13.9 μmol/L

5) Complete Blood Cell Count Test (CBC): Also known as Full Blood Count or Full Blood Exam test. The cells in our circulatory system are primarily categorized into three major types: White Blood Cells (Leukocytes), Red Blood Cells (Erythrocytes) and Platelets (Thrombocytes). An unusually high or low number of these cells may be symptomatic of many forms of diseases. This is what a typical CBC test looks like:

Component Standard Range

White Blood Cells 4.0 - 11.0 K/μL
Red Blood Cells 44 - 6.0 M/μL
Hemoglobin 13.5 - 18.0 g/dL
Hematocrit 40.0 - 52.0 %
MCV 80.0 - 100.0 fL
MCH 27.0 - 33.0 pg
MCHC 31.0 - 36.0 g/dL
RDW < 16.4 %
Platelet Count 150 - 400 K/μL
Neutrophil 49 - 64 %
Neutrophil Bands 0 - 10 %
Lymphocyte 26 - 46 %
Monocyte 0 - 12 %
Eosinophil 0 - 5 %
Basophil 0 - 2 %

6) Factor V (Leiden) Mutation: This is an inherited disorder of blood clotting. Factor V Leiden is the name of a particular genetic alteration that results in thrombophilia, meaning a higher tendency to form blood clots in the blood vessels. People who have the Factor V Leiden Mutation are at somewhat higher risk of clot formation. The clots can develop in the large veins in the legs called Deep Venous Thrombosis (DVT). The clots can also travel in the bloodstream and embed themselves in the lungs. It results in blockage of the main artery of the lungs or one of its branches. This condition is called Pulmonary Embolism (PE). The standard range for this test should be NEGATIVE.

7) Factor II Mutation: It is another type of genetic risk factor that doubles or even triples the possibility of clot formation in the veins. This variant is commonly related to both deep vein thrombosis and pulmonary embolism. The standard range for this test should be NEGATIVE as well.

8) Systemic Lupus Erythematosus (SLE) Panel: It is a test done to detect symptoms of an autoimmune disease in which the immune system of an individual inadvertently attacks the healthy tissues and cells. The causes of autoimmune diseases are not entirely known and more research is going on in this connection. Almost everyone with SLE develops joint pain and swelling. Some people even develop arthritis. However, SLE is closely associated with the brain and central nervous system as well. Indications like seizures, blood clots, numbness, tingling, and headaches are some of the possible aftereffects of SLE.

The standard Range is NEGATIVE, meaning all the component results in this test should be negative.

9) Protein S Antigen: A disorder in Protein S Antigen correlates closely with increased risk of blood clot formation in the veins (Venous Thrombosis). Here are the various components of this test:

Component Standard Range

Protein S Free 57 - 171 %

Protein S Antigenic 70 - 140 %

10) Protein C Antigen: It is a rear genetic disorder and a Protein C deficiency correlates with increased risk of Venous Thrombosis. Here are the typical values for this test:

Component Standard Range

Protein C Antigen 70 - 140 %

11) Activated Protein C Resistance: Activated Protein C Resistance (APCR) is a type of Hemostatic disorder (a procedure that causes bleeding to stop within a damaged blood vessel). Either it can be acquired or it can be hereditary. Its unusual range means there is an inadequate anticoagulant response to Activated Protein C. Also, this disorder can result in increased risk of Venous Thrombosis, and that can lead to problems with blood circulation. For example, it can cause pulmonary embolism. Here is the normal range for this test:

Component Standard Range

APC Resistance - Greater than or equal to 2.1

12) Protein S Activity: The deficiency of Protein S can also result in blood clotting and individuals deficient in Protein S can develop unusual blood clots. A mild deficiency in Protein S can lead to Deep Vein Thrombosis (DVT) of the arms and legs. Moreover, if it travels through the blood vessels and is stuck in the lungs, a life-threatening situation such as pulmonary embolism can arise. Here is the normal range of Protein S Activity:

Component Standard Range

Protein S 65 - 140 %

13) Protein C Activity: Protein C also plays a significant role in monitoring anticoagulation and maintain the pervious nature of the blood vessel walls. Here is the normal range of this test:

Component Standard Range

Protein C 70 - 130 %

14) Erythrocyte Sedimentation Rate (ESR): It is a blood test that measures and monitors inflammation in the body. This test estimates the speed with which the red blood cells in a tube of blood fall to the bottom of the tube. Here is the standard range of this test:

Component Standard Range

Sedimentation Rate 0 - 15 mm/hr

15) CK (Creatine Kinase) Muscle Enzyme: This test is performed to determine the inflammation of the muscles. It can also be performed to know any muscle damage such as weakness of the muscles, muscle pain, etc. Here is the standard range of this test:

Component Standard Range

Creatine Kinase 39 - 308 U/L

16) Antithrombin III Activity (AT3): This is a type of protein that controls blood clotting. Lower than normal Antithrombin III means that you are at an increased risk of blood clotting. It happens if there is no AT3 in your blood or AT3 is not functioning properly. The normal range for this test is:

Component Standard Range

Antithrombin III 80 - 120 %

17) ANA (Anti Nuclear Antibody) Screen with

Reflex Titler and Pattern: This is another test like the one SLE Panel test mentioned in point 8 earlier. The purpose of this test is to evaluate a patient for any autoimmune disorders that can affect many tissues and organs in the body. The normal range for this test is:

Component Standard Range
ANA Screen NEGATIVE

Chapter 8

How to Treat a Stroke Patient

The treatment of a stroke depends on the type of stroke. There are different treatment methods for the ischemic stroke / TIA and hemorrhagic stroke. The treatment plan also depends on some other factors like, how much time has passed since the symptoms began and if you have some other severe or moderate medical conditions. For example, if you have preexisting conditions, allergies to various drugs, your age and general health.

Remember, strokes (whether ischemic / TIAs or hemorrhagic) are medical emergencies and need immediate attention. If you feel you are having a stroke, and it is impacting your motor skills, call 911 in the USA. In the UK call 999 and in the European Union call 122, otherwise call the applicable emergency services number for your country of residence.

If you feel some numbness of arms and legs, do not drive to the hospital under any circumstance. Let someone else drive you to the Emergency Room. Do not even walk to a medical facility if it is at a stone throw distance from your residence. Remember, if you live in a place that has very high humidity, you will dehydrate yourself and dehydration during a stroke can further exacerbate your condition. As the brain is made up of approximately 75% water, dehydration during a stroke reduces the percentage of water to the brain and does even more damage.

All right, so once you receive the initial treatment from paramedics, you will be transported to the nearest hospital in case the stroke paralyzes you. The doctor will start the treatment, evaluate your history, and help you in preventing any further complications.

Now, let us go into the treatment of various types of stroke.

Treating Ischemic Attack and TIA:

The ischemic stroke and TIA, as mentioned earlier, are the most common types of stroke. So I am going to cover it first.

The treatment for an ischemic stroke or TIA can be done through medicines, medical procedures, or a combination of both. For example, if you had an ischemic stroke, and you were transported to the hospital within four hours, the doctor might inject a clot buster drug into your vein. This medicine is called **tPA** (Tissue Plasminogen Activator). This drug breaks up the blood clots in the arteries of the brain.

However, if you have a medical condition where tPA cannot be administered, the doctor might give you some blood-thinning medicine. For example, aspirin can be given to prevent the platelets from clustering together to form new blood clots. Eventually, as a long-term treatment, the doctor might recommend some blood-thinning medicines like Warfarin, Pradaxa, Xarelto or Eliquis. These drugs will help you in preventing new clot formation and ensuring that the existing blood clots either dissolve completely or do not get larger.

Besides the medicines, some medical procedures also might be recommended to you if necessary.

The doctor might recommend a procedure called Carotid Endarterectomy (CEA) in case he finds a major plaque buildup. The plaque could have formed in either your left or the right carotid artery or maybe both the arteries. During this procedure, the surgeon will make an incision or an opening in the neck to access the carotid arteries and remove the plaque buildup in them. This procedure restores the normal flow of oxygen-rich blood. This surgery is extremely helpful for people who have narrow or blocked carotid arteries. It even lowers the risk of getting a stroke in patients without any stroke symptoms yet.

There is another procedure called Carotid Angioplasty for treating the carotid artery disease. In this procedure, a balloon is inflated to push the plaque outward against the wall of the artery. Once this is completed, the doctor then places a small metal stent in the artery to prevent the artery from being blocked again.

However, a surgeon who is very experienced with these

types of procedures should perform the Carotid Angioplasty. Although the surgery is relatively safe if done by qualified surgeons, serious complications can occur including another stroke or death during this procedure. Therefore, it is better to talk to a renowned surgeon and understand the associated risks and benefits.

There have been some advances in some alternate medical treatments recently for treating ischemic strokes. I am going to cover two such treatment options.

Intra-arterial Thrombolysis (IAT): In this procedure, the doctor inserts a long flexible tube called a catheter into the groin area of the patient that goes all the way to the tiny arteries of the brain. The surgeon then delivers specific medicines like Urokinase, Streptokinase, Prourokinase, etc. through this catheter to break blood clots in the brain.

MERCI Retriever: The second recent treatment option is caller MERCI Retriever. MERCI stands for Mechanical Embolus Removal in Cerebral Ischemia. The MERCI Retriever was designed by the University of California, Los Angeles in 2001. This device is used for removing the blood clots from an artery. During this procedure, a catheter is inserted into the affected area of the brain through the carotid artery. Then the blood clot is pulled out through the catheter. MERCI retriever is different from IAT; the blood clots are pulled out from the affected area of the brain. While as in an IAT procedure, the blood clots are broken into small pieces in the affected area of the brain.

Now let us talk about the different treatment plans for treating the hemorrhagic stroke.

Hemorrhagic Stroke Treatment:

As noted in the previous chapters, the hemorrhagic stroke occurs if a blood vessel leaks blood in the brain or if a blood vessel ruptures in the brain. When a patient experiences a hemorrhagic stroke, the first step in the treatment process by the doctor is to control the bleeding along with finding the cause of bleeding in the brain. It is imperative to keep in mind that blood-thinning medicines cannot treat a hemorrhagic stroke, as these medications will make the bleeding even worse.

One of the leading causes of a hemorrhagic stroke is high blood pressure. And here is why it is so. The arteries carry oxygenated blood from the heart to different parts of the body. Smaller arteries called arterioles are smaller diameter blood vessels that extend and branch out from the main arteries and branches out further into capillaries. The main arteries like the aorta that come out of the heart, the coronary arteries that go to the heart, and the carotid arteries that go to the neck are much thicker. These arteries can withstand blood pressure at higher levels.

The problem occurs mainly in the capillaries. They are extremely fragile and narrow, and they branch out from the mini arteries to various parts of the body. If a person is suffering from high blood pressure for a long time, it is likely that the thin and extremely delicate capillaries in the brain might burst open. From that point forward, they will leak blood into the brain due to high blood pressure. However, that does not mean as we learned earlier that the blood could not leak in the arteries as well due to plaque buildup.

Sometimes a surgery might be needed as a last resort for treating the hemorrhagic stroke. Some of the surgical procedures are Aneurysm Clipping, Coil Embolization, and Arteriovenous Malformation repair. Let us learn more about each of these procedures one by one:

Aneurysm Clipping: It's a surgical procedure performed to treat an aneurysm. Over a period, if left undetected and untreated the aneurysm can become thin and weak. If the person is suffering from high blood pressure, the aneurysm can burst open or start leaking blood in the brain resulting in a subarachnoid hemorrhage. To prevent this from happening, the neurosurgeon makes a small incision in the brain. Then a tiny clamp is placed at the base or the neck of the aneurysm to block the normal flow of blood in the balloon. These clips are made of titanium and remain in the affected area permanently. This procedure is done under general anesthesia, and the patient has to stay in the hospital for several days under intensive care.

Coil Embolization: This procedure is somewhat less complicated as the neurosurgeon does not have to place an incision in the brain. Instead, a catheter is inserted through the groin into an artery all the way to the exact location of the aneurysm. Then a tiny coil is pushed through the tube all the way to the aneurysm. This small coil produces a blood clot at the neck of the aneurysm and prevents any blood flow into the balloon and then preventing the bursting of the balloon. This procedure is also done in a hospital under general anesthesia, and the patient has to be monitored for several days in an intensive care unit.

Arteriovenous Malfunction Repair (AVM): An AVM is a tangle or a knot of abnormal blood vessels connecting the arteries and veins in the brain. A direct connection between one or more arteries and the veins can result in many complications. Some serious problems can occur as the veins are generally thin-walled, and they cannot accept high-pressure blood flow for an extended timeframe. That situation can result in the AVM getting ruptured in the brain and bleeding to start.

A small percentage of people (less than 1%) are born with brain or spinal cord AVM (congenital). Few people can develop it at a later part of their lives. However, one good thing is that AVMs are not hereditary, meaning they are not passed from parents to children. A CT scan or an MRI detects the AVM. Once detected, an angiogram is done in which a special contrast in injected into the blood vessels of the brain. The angiogram precisely pinpoints the location of the AVM and the surrounding arteries. Next, the doctor performs the AVM repair procedure. The AVM repair helps in preventing any further complications of bleeding in the brain.

There are three main methods where the neurosurgeon can repair the AVM. They are as follows:

1) Endovascular Embolization: In this procedure, a catheter is inserted in the groin area all the way into the arteries in the brain to the AVM and then a drug is inserted into these arteries. This procedure shuts off the artery and reduces the blood flow through the AVM. Endovascular Embolization is a preparatory step in treating the AVM, as it does not completely get rid of the AVM. The doctor might recommend either Microsurgical Resection or Stereotactic Radiotherapy as a more effective cure for the AVM.

2) Microsurgical Resection: This is the standard and most well-known procedure for treating AVM. During Microsurgical Resection, a part of the bone from the skull is removed to expose the brain. This process is called craniotomy in medical terms. After that, the AVM is detached from the brain or the spinal cord using a microscope.

3) Stereotactic Radiotherapy: In this procedure a highly concentrated dose of radiation beams are focused on the core of the AVM in one session. The treatment cycle runs very slowly. In fact, over a period of 2 to 5 years, the blood vessels of the AVM shrink and the AVM closes down.

These were various treatment options for stroke. Besides this, the doctor might also recommend lifestyle changes to treat future stroke risk factors. They lifestyle changes are called as modified factors for stroke treatment and prevention. These are some tips and techniques that are totally in your control. If you incorporate them into your daily life, it will help you in preventing another stroke in conjunction with medicines. This topic will be covered in the next chapter.

Chapter 9

How to Prevent Another Stroke in the Near Future

In order to treat the risk factors of having another stroke, you will have to make drastic lifestyle changes in your day-to-day life. After a stroke, you might go in a state of denial and shock. You might think what if there is a recurrence of stroke. So reinforce positive thoughts in yourself every day. After all, it was a thing of the past, and now you need to look forward. It is your outlook toward life that plays a big role here. If you maintain this attitude, you will regain your health at a much faster rate.

You should not stay alone for a long time because you might go into a state of deep thought and even become despondent or apprehensive about your future. Your spouse should spend as much time as possible with you and engage you in a positive, interactive and inspirational conversation. For example, talking about stroke survivors and telling you how these tough people fought with this illness audaciously. These inspiring stories will give you hope and reasons to live and face these tough moments.

Watch funny and inspirational TV shows, videos on

the internet and listen to inspirational audios. It will have an incredible impact on your disposition. Moreover, it has been rightly said that laughter is the best medicine.

Another way that could help you heal faster is to stay in a different place or city for some time. Especially a place that is full of natural beauty or a place that has spiritual significance. Even a place where you would have dreamed of living or would have considered an ideal location to live and move in your lifetime. However, your family has to take a decision and consider all the pros and cons of moving to the new place temporarily. Particularly your spouse has to make this important choice.

On the other hand, there is a caveat though. If you already have had multiple strokes in the past, then moving from your current residence may not work in all the scenarios. Because multiple strokes result in dramatic changes in the brain's anatomy including the individual's thinking capabilities and his responses to various stimuli. Therefore, a change of place may not matter to you in such a situation. Patients who have had multiple strokes often remain detached from worldly affairs and they often resist frequent moves to different places.

Keep yourself busy with brain games and puzzles. Besides strengthening the cognitive skills, they will keep you engaged. You will think less about your illness.

Regular follow-ups with the doctors and giving them updates should be the norm. Stop smoking as smoking can damage the blood vessels and raise your risk of having another stroke. You should even avoid being a passive smoker. A passive smoker is one who is present frequently in an area where other individuals smoke. Similarly lose weight if you are overweight. Target a Body Mass Index (BMI) of less than 25. BMI is a measure of your weight in correlation to your height. It will give you an estimate of the total body fat. A BMI between 25 and 29.9 is considered overweight, and a BMI of more than 30 is considered obese.

Follow a healthy diet. Choose lots of fruits and vegetable along with whole grain products. Healthy foods are one that are low in saturated fats, trans fats, and cholesterol. Cut down drastically on your sugar intake and completely stop consuming soda and energy drinks. Similarly choose foods that are low in sodium as too much salt can raise your blood pressure. If you drink alcoholic beverages either quit drinking altogether or drink in moderation.

Maintain a highly active lifestyle. If you exercise on a regular basis, you will be able to control high blood pressure, high cholesterol, maintain your weight and manage your stress level. Purchase a premium blood pressure monitor and keep logs of the results for record keeping. Numerous smartphone apps can be used for record keeping. However, before you start any exercise plan, it is always recommended to talk to your doctor about it. Moderate exercise of one hour a day and three days a week is more than enough to keep you in good shape. However, immediately consult your neurologist if you see some unusual symptoms while exercising.

Individuals who had a stroke due to cerebral thrombosis, their doctor might recommend taking a baby aspirin (81mg) once a day to reduce the risk of another stroke. It reduces the risk but does not necessarily mean eliminating the possibility of another stroke. If you have high cholesterol, the doctor might also recommend a medicine for reducing the cholesterol. Similarly, if you have hypertension, blood pressure lowering medication might be prescribed as well.

Likewise, individuals who had a stroke due to cerebral embolism, the doctors might recommend anticoagulant drugs. The anticoagulant drugs reduce the risk of clot formation in the brain. The most commonly prescribed drug is called Warfarin.

Start a daily practice of meditation. It will calm your mind and address your emotional challenges after having a stroke. You will feel relaxed, get better sleep, reduce stress, and improve your mental faculty.

Chapter 10

How Does a Person's Life Change After a Major Stroke

Once the patient stabilizes after a stroke, he is discharged from the hospital. The patient can then return home with the support of a general practitioner, family members, a community care team (social worker), etc.

After a major stroke, the patient's life changes drastically. Here are some physiological, emotional, psychological, and mental changes you can expect to notice in the patient. These changes may become apparent immediately or after a few weeks. Sometimes it may take several months, or even more than a year, to notice dramatic biological changes in the patient.

Paralysis: If a person suffers a major stroke suddenly, it will paralyze his body on either the left or right side, or below the waist. It can also result in a partial paralysis, such as a facial paralysis. If there is a complete paralysis on the right side of the body, it means that the left hemisphere of the brain has been damaged. Naturally, the person will be confined to the bed until some level of recovery is achieved. However, if the individual has had multiple strokes, and with each stroke he is recovering one step but deteriorating two steps, the situation becomes commiserative.

Having said that, here is what a stroke patient would feel about himself after paralysis of his body. Let us say he paralyzes his right arm and right leg after a stroke. First of all, the field of vision facing the affected side of the body may be diminished in some patients. For the first few days after the body becomes paralyzed, he will try his best to get up or move his limbs while lying down on the bed. You can see from his facial expressions how hard he is attempting to move his arm or leg. After some time, he will just give up trying to lift his arm or leg, as he knows that it is not going to help.

The patient will also try to sleep on the paralyzed side of his body, and here is the reason: If you turn him in the opposite direction, he will feel an acute numbness of the paralyzed side of his body, as if that part of the body is virtually nonexistent. After a while, he will either turn around and sleep on his back, or will again turn towards the paralyzed side of his body.

Extreme care should be taken not to pull the paralyzed arm while lifting the patient from a bed, as it will result in dislocation of the shoulder. This would create further complications of the shoulder joint and the neck. You can also put a pillow under the affected arm for comfort. Likewise, a pillow can be placed between the legs if one leg is paralyzed as well.

Shock and state of denial: Immediately after a stroke, the patient will be in a state of shock and self-denial for some days. He will start thinking negative thoughts, such as, "why me", "why so soon", "why now" etc. Gradually, the patient will have a realization that his situation is for real, and he will transition from a state of denial to a state of acceptance. This time around, you can play a prominent role as a family member. You need to remind the patient that whatever has happened cannot be undone. So the best thing to do is to forget about the stroke incident and focus on an aggressive treatment plan.

Acute pain and numbness: This is one of the topics in this chapter that requires special thoughtfulness. After a major stroke, an individual experiences chronic pain in the affected areas. For example, if a person paralyzes his right arm and right leg, he will suffer shooting pain in the neck and shoulder joint. While the person is lying down on his back, try to slowly raise his right arm upwards. You will notice an immediate reaction on his face due to acute pain and suffering. If the person has not lost his voice, he might even scream due to intense pain while you are holding his arm upwards.

The condition becomes pitiable when the patient cannot speak, and you are trying to raise his paralyzed arm toward the headboard of the bed. You will notice facial expressions of extreme discomfort. The patient will not scream, as he has lost his voice. Due to paralysis, normal blood circulation is not happening in the arm, which eventually results in muscle atrophy as well.

Never pull the patient's arm or try to rotate it. Any sudden movement or stretch in the arm can lead to shoulder and joint dislocation. Ask a physical therapist or a neurologist how to handle the arms and legs of the patient so that there is no further damage to the muscles and joints.

Thinking/Cognitive Deficit: After a major stroke, most of the people wonder what happened to their cognitive skills and motor skills so suddenly. People who are deep thinkers and highly emotional are more likely to go into a heavy thought process and continue thinking, compared to people who ruminate less or people who are gregarious. Besides, sociable people tend to express their feelings to family and friends or divert their attention to other things.

Therefore, individuals who are deep thinkers, and who are either introverts or ambiverts need special care after a stroke. Family members have to encourage them continually, inspire them, and keep them positive. Exceptional care should be taken not to hurt the feelings of the patient or talk negatively about anything. As a caregiver, try to show equanimity and be stoic in front of the patient as much as you can.

Keep a log of how the patient's thinking is doing and report any unusual patterns to the neurologist or the psychologist. Remember, the thinking and the mood of the patient have to be monitored on a regular basis. If left unchecked and untreated, here is what might happen: If a person has had a fearless personality, always shown tenacity and enthusiasm, the gradual changes that take place in the individual's brain after a major stroke can make him an entirely opposite person. Now that person will be more careful about visiting the bathroom to avoid a fall. He may want to be close to the family members all the time. He might start getting apprehensive about trivial things or want to sleep most of the time. He may get palpitations, complain shortness of breath, become eccentric or keep saying illogical things.

Sometimes he might even have delusions like scarcity of resources, even though he might have resources in abundance whether money, paraphernalia and so forth. In this situation, the family members, spouse in particular, are unable to fathom as to what happened to their loved one all of a sudden. Their disparity and worry are justifiable as in most of the cases they have no clue about the level of damage to the patient's brain.

Physical Energy: A stroke diminishes an individual's physical energy and if not addressed on time can have far-reaching implications on the patient's physique. It is imperative for the patient to do physical therapy and exercise to avoid muscular atrophy and prevent bedsores. There will be instances when the patient may not listen to you or the physical therapist due to a mood swing or pain. During these times, you have to show an enormous amount of patience and work with him with compassion and care.

However, things can get tough if the patient has had multiple strokes and is unable to respond to the commands due to dementia or memory loss. In that case, you may have to exercise the patient's limbs manually and work with a qualified physical therapist. As mentioned earlier, the patient will experience extreme level of pains when you stretch the shoulder muscles. So handle his arms and legs with care.

Emotional energy: The patient will feel significantly disturbed emotionally. He will start feeling sad and vent out his emotions from time to time by his facial expressions, moist eyes or tears. He might have regrets about things he would have liked to do in life that he cannot do anymore. Put yourself in his shoes to understand his feelings. Give so much love and make him realize that the whole family cares for him. Give empowerment and tell the person (if his cognitive skills are somewhat okay) that we are in this all together.

Talk less: The patient will gradually talk less (unless he has lost his faculty of speech) as the time progresses and keep thinking most of the time. Make sure to engage the person in interactive and quality conversations. Talk about jokes and funny anecdotes. Ask open-ended questions so that the patient answers in sentences and chunks of words. If you ask close-ended questions, he will only respond by saying yes or no.

Compose your thoughts and questions ahead of time so that you are in a position of asking smart questions. Besides that, try to vary your questions during the day. Do not repeat your questions. Ask questions about subjects that have been of interest to the patient. Rekindle some of the sweetest memories of the past with the patient.

Confusion and inability to understand: If an individual has suffered multiple strokes in the left brain, there is a possibility that the patient will have difficulty understanding things. He might get confused while trying to express himself, or when somebody tries to say something. This condition might improve over time if the patient does not suffer subsequently with more strokes. On the other hand, the condition might worsen if the individual keeps getting repeated strokes. It also holds true if the hippocampus of the brain gets impaired due to a stroke. In that case, the patient will lose his memory faculty as well.

Words may not come out even though he wants to say something. Sometimes the patient may wish to say something, but either forgets how to say it or does not know the words to say it. The situation becomes agonizing when you realize that the patient cannot talk but wants to say something just by looking at his facial expressions. As a caregiver, you need to have an innate power of observation and learn to understand the micro-expressions of the face. Read some books on body language and micro-expressions to understand what the patient might be trying to convey.

Irritable behavior and getting angry over small things: It is yet another symptom of stroke patients, especially if the patient is paralyzed and bed-ridden. As the patient is unable to perform his daily chores all by himself, he will gradually become desperate and indignant. Slowly this will translate into an irritable behavior. Sometimes he will start getting angry or irritated over trivial things. He may not cooperate with you or follow your instruction during an exercise session or while working with a physical therapist.

Sometimes the patient might inadvertently self-inflict an injury or hurt the caregiver. The patient might grab the caregiver's hair or squeeze her arm or hand. Therefore, it is safe for the caregiver to approach the patient from the paralyzed side of the body due to his weakness or lack of motor skills on that side. Try not to irritate the patient and show an enormous amount of compassion and patience. With practice as a caregiver, you will become cognizant of handling various tasks.

Bladder and bowel control: A major stroke can affect the normal functioning of the bladder and bowel movement. If the person is paralyzed, the doctor might recommend an internal catheter temporarily. However, the internal catheter should not be used for more than two weeks as it might result in urinary tract infections. If the patient can walk with support, encourage him to visit the bathroom frequently, as long as it is safe to do so. But if the patient has extensively impaired his motor skills due to multiple strokes, it is better to use a urine pot on the bed, empty it frequently and sanitize it after every use. At nighttime, the patient can wear an adult diaper as well.

Inability to swallow food - especially liquids: A major stroke might render the patient incapable of swallowing. In that case, the doctor will advise Nasogastric Intubation or NG tube. A small tube is inserted through one of the nostrils, past the throat, and all the way into the stomach. The patient is administered a measured liquid diet as recommended by a nutritionist. If the NG tube is to be used at home, follow the instructions from the doctor. If used incorrectly, the patient might get pulmonary aspiration (a condition in which food, liquids, saliva goes into the lungs) which can be dangerous. As the liquid diet is administered in small quantities, the caregiver will have to feed the patient more frequently.

Once the patient starts getting a little better, he will find the NG tube very irritating and will try to pull it out using the healthy arm. If that happens, there are chances of nasal bleeding and the anesthesiologist will have to insert a new tube in the other nostril. Inserting a nasal tube is extremely painful and irritating. If the patient is unable to swallow, the doctor has to thrust the tube and push it deep into the stomach through the esophagus. Sometimes the patient might scream due to a terrible irritation of the nasal passage. As an example, try to insert a twig or a grass blade in one of your nostrils. How will you feel? Within no time, you will start sneezing, and your eyes will get watery. Compare this scenario to the one in which a long tube is inserted into the nostril of a stroke patient all the way into his stomach and placed there for days and days.

The doctor will often recommend securing the healthy arm of the patient with the bedpost so that the patient does not try to pull the tube out from his nose. Give serious thought to this situation. How will the patient feel with one arm paralyzed, and the other arm tied with a cord? If he wants to scratch his body somewhere, what will he do? To make the situation even worse, what if the patient has lost his speech as well? He cannot even ask for help from a family member. He has to suffer silently for days and days.

Complete or partial loss of speech: We often take our health for granted without realizing the importance of each minor and major organ of our body. I will tell you a small incident. When my dad had a major stroke on June 29, 2012, he lost his speech, besides paralyzing the right side of his body. The swallowing function also got impacted. After around a week, he was shifted from an Intensive Care Unit (ICU) to a private room of the hospital. He would be administered a liquid diet by a nurse through the nasal tube along with some crushed medicines from time to time.

One day I was sitting on a chair reading a book. A few minutes later, two nurses gave a liquid diet to my dad, along with some medicines, and then left the room after a while. Around half an hour later, I noticed that my dad's facial expressions were showing signs of anguish and pain. I asked him whether he was all right, knowing that he would be unable to respond or talk. I was trying to figure out what could be wrong. I checked his posture, all the lines, the IV pole, and the pressure pads on the legs. Everything seemed to be all right. So I went back to my seat and continued reading my book while periodically looking at my dad's face.

It was an incident of déjà vu. As an afterthought, it just

stuck in my mind to turn him to the left side. While I was doing that, I noticed the nurse had accidentally left the tube along with the attached plunger on the bed after they were done feeding liquid diet and medicines to my dad. While lying down on his back, my dad's back was pressing against the plastic tube that had a sharp rim. The tube plunger attachment had created a wound in his back and blood was oozing out from that area.

I promptly removed the tube, and then called the nurse to apply some medicine and tape the wound. In a few minutes, I noticed that dad was trying to say something to me but was unable to do so. His facial expressions were a little different now. I could see he was feeling very relieved by observing micro-expressions on his face. I learned a big lesson, and understood the importance of speech even more. I thought if my dad were able to talk, he would have told me instantly that something was hurting his back. I was feeling powerless deep inside and trying to reconcile with the realities.

Dysphagia: This is a medical term for a symptom in which a patient is unable to swallow. If a stroke affects the esophagus of the patient, then he may have difficulty swallowing or chewing food. It often happens in tandem with the loss of speech functionality. With physical therapy, it is possible to regain this faculty of chewing and swallowing food.

Aphasia: This is a medical term for a symptom in which a stroke patient partially or completely loses the ability to articulate ideas or comprehend spoken and written languages. The patient might sometimes say a word or two, which might sometimes make sense to family members. However, if the brain damage is extensive, then the patient may not be able to comprehend anything or respond to any external stimulus.

In the case of my dad, who knew six languages, there were moments in the hospital and at home when sometimes he was unable to respond to our conversation or would feel confused. Compare it with happy times when he would converse in different languages, write incredible stories and tell wonderful anecdotes. But the strokes wiped out all those wonderful memories in no time. What a reversal of fortune for a person so full of life and enthusiasm.

Nevertheless, if the damage to the brain is not extensive, and the patient has not had repeated strokes, aphasia can get better with time through treatment and following the expert advice of doctors and therapists.

Chapter 11

How to Arrange Treatment and Home Care for a Stroke Patient

In this chapter, I am going to talk about things you will need at home to attend to the stroke patient's needs. This chapter will also give some insight into the mental and emotional states of caregivers and how to manage their daily lives.

Here are some of the things you will need to arrange for the stroke patient:

Bed: A paralyzed stroke patient will need a reclining bed at home. Sometimes you will have to recline the patient's bed forward so she may eat in a sitting position. Other times she may just want to sit on the bed for some time in a sitting position. The bed can either be an electrically reclining bed or a manually reclining bed. With a manually reclining bed, you will have to turn the handlebar manually, either clockwise or counterclockwise, to raise the bed or lay it flat.

Air mattress: This is one of the most indispensable items for the patient. Due to her inability to move and shift in the bed with ease, there are greater chances of the patient getting bedsores on her body. Moreover, if the bedsores increase rapidly in number and size, it can be life-threatening. Therefore, an air mattress is a solution to the problem. The air mattress gets inflated with an attached pump, and the mattress itself has interlaced air pockets. One channel gets inflated, and the other channel gets deflated. After a few minutes, the operation reverses. The inflated channel deflates, and the deflated channel inflates. In this manner, an uneven pressure is applied to the patient's body, especially her back, which prevents bedsores.

Special chair: You might need a sturdy chair that can recline so the patient can sometimes sit on it. Do not seat the patient on a chair with castor wheels, as it can slide or shift and cause injuries.

Physical Therapist: You might have to find a qualified physical therapist who will visit the patient at home. Physical therapy is needed to strengthen the affected muscles and tissues to regain partial or complete strength. You may have to refer to the health insurance provider for benefits and eligibility for the patient.

Occupational Therapist: Check with the doctor if the patient needs the help of an occupational therapist. An occupational therapist can assist the patient in activities important to her on a daily basis, such as eating, dressing, hobbies, and her professional activities. An occupational therapist also has adequate knowledge and training to work with people who have a mental illness or emotional problems, such as depression, mood swings and extreme levels of stress common in stroke patients.

Speech and Language Therapist: If the individual has lost her voice or her voice has been impaired due to a major stroke, then you might have to work with a speech therapist as well. The speech therapist can help the patient to regain her speech and heal her voice box.

Nutritionist: A nutritionist will help you in advising the dietary needs of the patient. The patient will have to follow strict dietary requirements as recommended by the nutritionist. It is even more important if the patient is unable to swallow due to a stroke. In that case, the nutritionist might recommend a liquid diet including the patient's daily nutritional requirements to be administered through the nasal tube.

Clinical Psychologist: As a family caregiver, you may want to consult a clinical psychologist to address the psychological needs of the patient.

Roles of family and relatives: The family members (spouse in particular) have to prepare themselves for a long and often difficult period ahead. It would be a good idea to talk to an experienced doctor or a psychologist to understand your roles and responsibilities better. You can also talk to families who have a stroke patient at home and ask questions about caregiving.

Support services in the community or stroke clubs: I would highly recommend that the patient join a stroke club. It is one of the best ways for the patient to regain hope and confidence by interacting with stroke survivors. When the patient listens to the incredible stories of stroke survivors or other patients in the club, it gives a big boost to the patient's mental and emotional health. Therefore, it will help the patient heal faster.

Full-time nurse: You may also consider hiring a full-time nurse to take care of the essential needs of the patient, especially if the patient is paralyzed and bedridden. It will decrease the workload of the family members to some extent. This is particularly applicable in the case of older patients, as their spouses will not be able to do certain things due to their old age and physical weakness. However, a lot depends on the willpower of the spouse as well. I have seen cases where spouses in their 60s and 70s have shown so much grit and dedication attending to the daily needs of their spouses that it sometimes brings youngsters to shame.

Feeding: If the patient is paralyzed on the dominant side of her body, she may not be willing to eat with her other hand. Therefore, as a family member or as a caregiver, you will initially have to feed her from time to time. However, after some time and with a little bit of practice, it is highly recommended to encourage the patient to eat by herself. You should also encourage the patient to try eating with the paralyzed hand as well in case it has started gaining some traction. It will ensure that her brain gets trained to use her weak hand slowly but steadily.

Dressing: If the patient is partially or completely paralyzed, you may have to learn about the best and safest ways to dress up the patient. Since the patient may not be in a position to balance her body, roll over on the bed, or stand up by herself, you need to be very creative in such a situation. If you try to support the person in the wrong way to lift her from the bed or a chair, you may hurt your back, shoulders, arms or your wrists. If you continue this practice, you might get some health issues later on. This is especially true for the spouse, especially if the spouse is old and frail. Get some tips from the doctor or the physical therapist about the correct ways of supporting the patient.

Washing and Bathing: Extreme care should be taken when giving a sponge bath or a shower to the stroke patient. There are significant chances of accidents happening in the bathroom. For example, the patient could have a fall, hit her head against a hard surface, or fracture a limb, etc. Once is a while you may let the patient sit on a stable chair in the bathtub and gently give her a shower. However, giving a shower in the bathroom may not be a viable option in many cases due to certain risks of being injured. A better option would be to give a sponge bath to the patient while using some antibiotic or antiseptic lotions.

Transfers - the ability to change from bed to a chair: The best way to move the patient from a bed to a chair is to tell the patient to bend her legs first. Then she should try to place her feet firmly on the floor and lean a little forward. If the patient cannot do it herself, then you may have to do the above procedure yourself. Once the patient bends forward, a major part of the body weight will shift on her legs. Then all you have to do is lift the patient gently from behind while keeping your back straight. A similar procedure can be applied while transferring the patient from a chair to the bed.

Standing and walking gear: You might need a walking cane or a walker to help the patient during physical therapy or while she is trying to take some steps either with assistance or by herself. Remember that too much sitting is bad even for an average healthy person.

Going to the toilet: Ensure the patient's room has an attached bathroom or the bathroom is not too far away. You may want to consider a bathroom with a wide doorframe for convenience. Another option would be to buy a portable toilet with a removable toilet bowl for a patient who is unable to walk.

Bladder function: If the patient has had multiple strokes in the past, it is difficult to control the bladder function in certain situations. In that case, make sure the patient goes to the bathroom after every two to three hours, even if she may not have any urge to urinate. A family member's help might be needed to take the patient to the bathroom.

Alternatively, you may help the patient to sit on a portable toilet seat several times a day. Extreme care should be taken not to put the patient on the toilet seat for too long, as it might damage the leg muscles and nerves due to prolonged compression.

Irregular bowel movement: If a person is paralyzed and is unable to move freely by herself, chances are the patient might occasionally become constipated. The solution would be to give plenty of fluids and provide food rich in fiber. For example, whole-wheat cereals, brown bread, fresh fruits and vegetables, salads, etc.

Stressful aspects of caring: After a person has had a stroke, there are chances the patient might have a rapid recovery (say within a few weeks to a few months). In such a scenario, things are not going to be that difficult for the family members. However, if the stroke is severe or a person has suffered from multiple strokes and is paralyzed, the chances are that the stroke patient may not fully recover even after getting the best treatment and best care. Her condition might even worsen with time. As expected, the patient will be completely dependent on family members for caregiving. Therefore, the immediate family members will have to cope with a tough time ahead.

Family members will have a feeling of regret and self-denial. Apart from the patient, they will get desperate and flabbergasted as to how their life changed all of a sudden. Initially, they will come to terms with fate and attend to the patient's needs. As time passes, and doctors say it could be a long path to recovery, such as several years, sometimes the caregivers might start getting hopeless and turn pessimistic.

At times, they will get irritated and feel sorry for the patient and themselves. They might curse their destiny, but at the same time keep attending the patient. If the patient's care is important no matter what, then serve her without feeling embittered during those moments. Having an enormous amount of patience and a big smile on your face can do wonders. Avoid talking about anything negative in front of the patient and shower unconditional love to her. It might be tough initially, but with a little practice, things can be managed.

Remember, the patient is watching you, and if she finds you in pain and agony, she will feel guilty about it. That could have some far-reaching implications for everybody.

Respite care - giving a break to the family members: I have seen some family members virtually losing their sanity during the prolonged caregiving process. As it can immensely affect them physically, mentally, emotionally and monetarily, it is extremely crucial to give some respite from the daily routine to the primary caregiver. For example, the primary caregiver can take a mini break, spend some time in the countryside, and meditate there. Some other options could be taking a few yoga classes, exercising, listening to music, working on a hobby temporarily, reading an inspiring book and so on. It will boost the physical, mental and emotional energies of the primary caregiver.

Getting back to work: A young stroke survivor might want to get back to work after completing the treatment. However, before resuming work, it would be wise to ask the neurologist whether it would be safe to drive to work and what precautions need to be taken while driving. Talking to her supervisor at work in detail so both of them can set up mutual expectations would be another wise move.

Epilogue

I hope you found useful and practical information in this book. As you might have noticed, a lot of medical terms have been used in this book. Therefore, chances are that you might find it hard to commit all of the key concepts and terms to memory after you finish reading the book. That is why I highly recommend you read this book several times from beginning to end. This will help you in committing the material into your long-term memory. I would also recommend that you take notes and highlight important sentences and paragraphs for quick reference.

I want you to give your undivided attention to the book when you are reading it again. If it fills your mind with a sense of dread and pathos, it means that it has created an indelible imprint on your mind by understanding the predicaments of a stroke patient. You will realize how important it is to keep yourself aware of stroke and the catastrophic effects it can bring in people's lives and their families.

I wish you all the best for your continued success in your life's journey. And above all, I wish your health span and your life span to be the same.

About the Author

Arun Thaploo is a business coach, critical thinker, motivational speaker, and sales and marketing expert. His primary role has been in turning around businesses using technology, increasing revenues, and improving people's lives by organizing seminars and workshops on personality development, improving thinking, and creativity.

Arun is a voracious reader who has read thousands of books and has committed himself to lifelong learning. His other areas of interest include music, travel, health and fitness, adventure sports, gardening, and photography. As an ardent traveler, he has been to multiple countries and touched people's lives by understanding human values and emotions. He has a great passion for helping corporations and individuals to explore hidden talent and skills to lead a fulfilling and meaningful life. You can email him at arun@arunthaploo.com if the mood strikes you.

Other Title by the Author

This book will give you powerful and data-driven tips on how to achieve success in various areas of your life in the 21st century.

Here are some of the things that you will learn from this book:

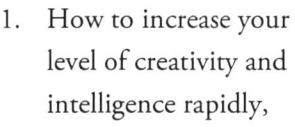

1. How to increase your level of creativity and intelligence rapidly, thereby making informed decision in life.
2. How to stay healthy by making incremental changes in your habits.
3. How to find a job in your chosen field quickly and how to rise to the top of the echelon in the company.
4. How to develop strong personal and professional relationships.
5. How to lead an amazing life after retirement. And much more.

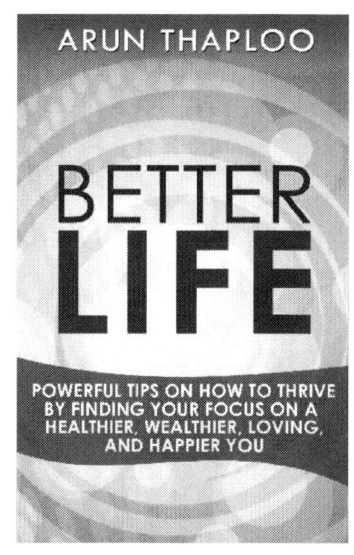

Urgent Plea

Thank you for purchasing this book. Please review this book on Amazon and share your thoughts on Facebook and Twitter. The more reviews I get for this book, more people will probably buy this book and read it. <u>Who knows, it might save somebody's life by espousing the contents of this book.</u>

I appreciate all your feedback and I would love to hear what you have to say. I need your opinion to create future books and products. So **PLEASE** leave a review on Amazon as I depend on your review to get the word out. You just have to write a few sentences and give a rating of your choice. You can come back later and write more if you wish. I will give a very honest look at all the reviews, both helpful reviews and critical reviews. That will help me immensely in bringing out a future update for this book including the latest research and advanced treatment options for stroke.

Printed in Poland
by Amazon Fulfillment
Poland Sp. z o.o., Wrocław